Beans and Grains Cookbook for Vegetarians

Harness the Benefits of Beans and Grains in Your Vegetarian Diet With Easy and Tasty Recipes

By
Linda Parker

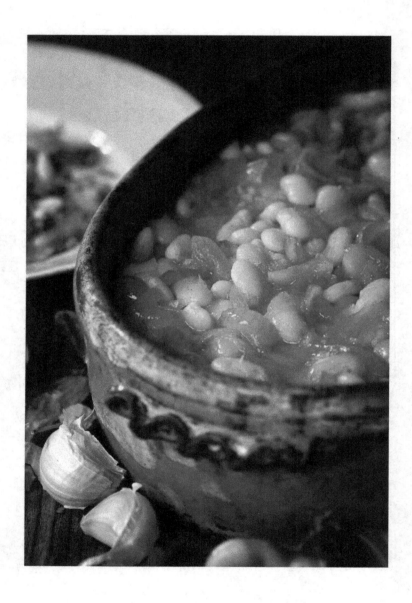

the publisher or the original author of this work can be in any fashion deemed liable for any hardship or damages that may befall them after undertaking information described herein.

Additionally, the information in the following pages is intended only for informational purposes and should thus be thought of as universal. As befitting its nature, it is presented without assurance regarding its prolonged validity or interim quality. Trademarks that are mentioned are done without written consent and can in no way be considered an endorsement from the trademark holder.

Table of Contents

Introduction

Vegetarianism refers to a lifestyle that excludes the consumption of all forms of meat including pork, chicken, beef, lamb, venison, fish, and shells. Depending on a person's belief and lifestyle, vegetarianism has different spectrums. There are vegetarians, who like to consume products that come from animals such as milk, eggs, cream and cheese. On the other end of that spectrum are the vegans. Vegans never consume meat or any product that comes from animals.

Benefits of Vegetarianism

According to research, living a vegetarian lifestyle lowers your risk of getting some of the major chronic diseases such as heart disease, cancer and type 2 diabetes. Vegetarians are 19 to 25% less likely to die of any kind of heart disease. The high consumption of fiber from grains also prevents the blood sugar spikes that lead to heart attacks and diabetes. The consumption of nuts, which are high in fiber, antioxidants and omega 3 fatty acids also helps lower the vegetarian's risk of getting heart attacks.

Due to the avoidance of red meat, you'll also eliminate a great deal of risk in getting certain types of cancer such as colon cancer. The high level of antioxidants from green leafy vegetables and fruits also helps in this area.

What About These Missing Nutrients?

Some people may be concerned with the lack of the following nutrients in a vegetarian diet however you'll find that there are certain types of vegetables and fruits that can supply these nutrients to give you a perfectly balanced diet. Some of the nutrients of concern are protein, iron, calcium and vitamin b12.

Protein can easily be found in beans and products made from beans such as tofu. Nuts and peas are also good sources of protein. Iron can also be found in tofu, beans, spinach, chard and cashews. Calcium can easily be found in soy milk, broccoli, collard greens, mustard greens and kale.

How to Make The Change

When you're starting out with this lifestyle, you might want to take baby steps. Start with 1 vegetarian meal per day. This allows you to adapt gradually to the different taste and flavors of a vegetarian diet. Once you're used to having a vegetarian meal every day, you can slowly add one more vegetarian meal until you've completely changed your lifestyle. Research has found that making small changes is more sustainable in the end. It's not a contest. Take your time and enjoy the different types of vegetarian meals. How To Use This Book As you browse through the pages, figure out which recipes you like and make them a part of your daily life. This book is filled with different types of vegan dishes and some of them include classic dishes that have been adapted to suit the vegan diet.

Red Bean Burrito Bowl with Chimichurri Sauce

Ingredients:
- 1 ancho chili, diced
- 1 red onion, diced
- 1 mild red chili, finely chopped
- 1 1/2 cup red beans
- 1 cup uncooked white rice
- 1 1/2 cups chopped tomatoes
- 1/2 cup water
- 4 tbsp. chimichurri sauce
- 1/2 tsp. cayenne pepper
- Sea salt
- Black pepper

Toppings:
- fresh coriander (cilantro), chopped spring onions, sliced avocado, guacamole, etc.

Directions:
1. Combine all the burrito bowl ingredients (not toppings) in a slow cooker.
2. Cook on low for 3 hours, or until the rice is cooked.
3. Serve hot with topping ingredients

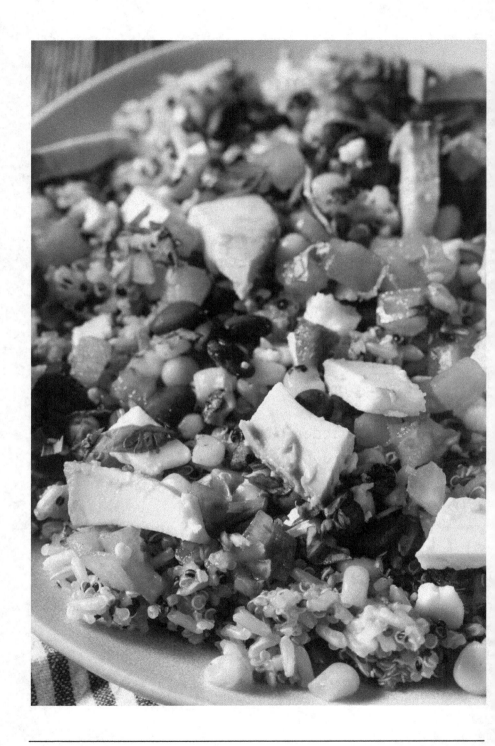

Black Rice Burrito Bowl with Vegan Chorizos

Ingredients:
- 5 Serrano peppers, diced
- 1 red onion, diced
- 1 mild red chili, finely chopped
- 1 1/2 cup navy beans, drained
- 1 cup uncooked black rice
- 1 1/2 cup chopped green tomatoes
- 1/2 cup water
- 1/4 cup vegan chorizos, coarsely chopped
- 1 tsp. dried thyme
- Sea salt
- Black pepper

Toppings:
- fresh coriander (cilantro), chopped spring onions, sliced avocado, guacamole, etc.

Directions:
1. Combine all the burrito bowl ingredients (not toppings) in a slow cooker.
2. Cook on low for 3 hours, or until the rice is cooked.
3. Serve hot with topping ingredients

Vegetarian Chimichurri Burrito Bowl

Ingredients:
- 1 red onion, diced or thinly sliced
- 1 green bell pepper (I used yellow), diced
- 1 mild red chili, finely chopped
- 1 ½ cups black beans, drained
- 1 cup Vegan Italian sausage, coarsely chopped
- 1 cup uncooked brown rice
- 1 ½ cups chopped tomatoes
- 1/2 cup water
- 4 tbsp. chimichurri sauce
- 1/2 tsp. cayenne pepper
- Sea salt
- Black pepper

Toppings:
- fresh coriander (cilantro), chopped spring onions, sliced avocado, guacamole, etc.

Directions:
1. Combine all the burrito bowl ingredients (not toppings) in a slow cooker.
2. Cook on low for 3 hours, or until the rice is cooked.
3. Serve hot with topping ingredients

Vegetarian Black Rice Burrito Bowl

Ingredients:
- 1 poblano chili, diced
- 1 red onion, diced
- 1 mild red chili, finely chopped
- 1 1/2 cup navy beans, drained
- 1 cup uncooked black rice
- 1 1/2 cup chopped green tomatoes
- 1/2 cup water
- 8 tbsp. pesto
- 1 tsp. Italian seasoning
- Sea salt
- Black pepper

Toppings:
- fresh coriander (cilantro), chopped spring onions, sliced avocado, guacamole, etc.

Directions:
1. Combine all the burrito bowl ingredients (not toppings) in a slow cooker.
2. Cook on low for 3 hours, or until the rice is cooked.
3. Serve hot with topping ingredients

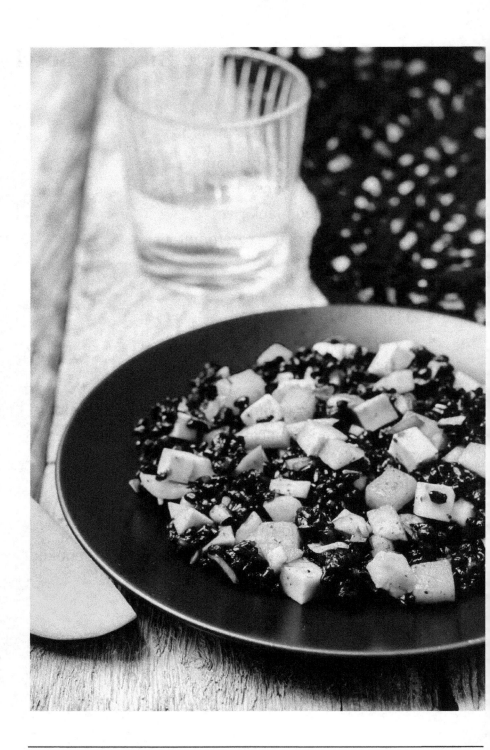

Brown Rice with Vegetarian Sausage and Black Bean Burrito Bowl

Ingredients:
- 5 jalapeno peppers, diced
- 1 red onion, diced
- 1 mild red chili, finely chopped
- 1 ½ cups black beans, drained
- 1 cup uncooked brown rice
- 1 ½ cups chopped tomatoes
- 1/2 cup water
- 1/4 cup vegetarian grain meat sausage (brand: Field Roast), coarsely chopped
- 1 tsp. dried thyme Sea salt Black pepper

Toppings:
- fresh coriander (cilantro), chopped spring onions, sliced avocado, guacamole, etc.

Directions:
1. Combine all the burrito bowl ingredients (not toppings) in a slow cooker.
2. Cook on low for 3 hours, or until the rice is cooked.
3. Serve hot with topping ingredients

Black Rice with Vegan Italian Sausage

Ingredients:
- 1 red onion, diced or thinly sliced
- 1 green bell pepper (I used yellow), diced
- 1 mild red chili, finely chopped
- 1 1/2 cup vegan Italian sausage, crumbled
- 1 cup uncooked black rice
- 1 1/2 cup chopped tomatoes
- 1/2 cup water
- 1/4 cup vegan chorizos, coarsely chopped
- 1 tsp. dried thyme
- Sea salt
- Black pepper

Toppings:
- fresh coriander (cilantro), chopped spring onions, sliced avocado, guacamole, etc.

Directions:
1. Combine all the burrito bowl ingredients (not toppings) in a slow cooker.
2. Cook on low for 3 hours, or until the rice is cooked.
3. Serve hot with topping ingredients

Brown Rice and Vegan Meatballs

Ingredients:
- 1 Anaheim pepper, diced
- 1 red onion, diced
- 1 mild red chili, finely chopped
- 1/2 cup meatless meatballs, crumbled
- 1 cup uncooked brown rice
- 1 ½ cups chopped tomatoes
- 1/2 cup water
- 4 tbsp. vegan cream cheese, sliced thinly
- 1 tsp. herbs de Provence
- Sea salt
- Black pepper

Toppings:
- fresh coriander (cilantro), chopped spring onions, sliced avocado, guacamole, etc.

Directions:
1. Combine all the burrito bowl ingredients (not toppings) in a slow cooker.
2. Cook on low for 3 hours, or until the rice is cooked.
3. Serve hot with topping ingredients

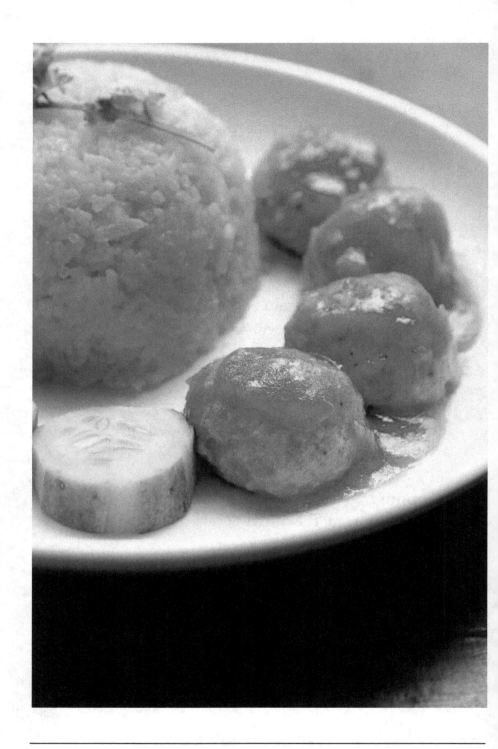

Chipotle Black Rice Burrito Bowl

Ingredients:
- 5 Serrano peppers, diced
- 1 red onion, diced
- 1 mild red chili, finely chopped
- 1 1/2 cup navy beans, drained
- 1 cup uncooked black rice
- 1 1/2 cup chopped tomatoes
- 1/2 cup water
- 1 tbsp chipotle hot sauce (or other favorite hot sauce)
- 1 tsp smoked paprika
- 1/2 tsp ground cumin
- Sea salt
- Black pepper

Toppings:
- fresh coriander (cilantro), chopped spring onions, sliced avocado, guacamole, etc.

Directions:
1. Combine all the burrito bowl ingredients (not toppings) in a slow cooker.
2. Cook on low for 3 hours, or until the rice is cooked.
3. Serve hot with topping ingredients

Pesto Brown Rice Burrito Bowl

Ingredients:
- 5 jalapeno peppers, diced
- 1 red onion, diced
- 1 mild red chili, finely chopped
- 1 ½ cups black beans, drained
- 1 cup uncooked brown rice
- 1 ½ cups chopped tomatoes
- 1/2 cup water
- 4 tbsp. pesto
- 1 tsp. Italian seasoning
- Sea salt
- Black pepper

Toppings:
- fresh coriander (cilantro), chopped spring onions, sliced avocado, guacamole, etc.

Directions:
1. Combine all the burrito bowl ingredients (not toppings) in a slow cooker.
2. Cook on low for 3 hours, or until the rice is cooked.
3. Serve hot with topping ingredients

Black Rice and Vegan Sausage Burrito Bowl

Ingredients:
- 1 red onion, diced or thinly sliced
- 1 green bell pepper (I used yellow), diced
- 1 mild red chili, finely chopped
- 1/2 cup vegetarian grain meat sausages, crumbled
- 1 cup uncooked black rice
- 1 1/2 cup chopped tomatoes
- 1/2 cup water
- 4 tbsp. vegan cream cheese, sliced thinly
- 1 tsp. herbs de Provence
- Sea salt
- Black pepper

Toppings:
- fresh coriander (cilantro), chopped spring onions, sliced avocado, guacamole, etc.

Directions:
1. Combine all the burrito bowl ingredients (not toppings) in a slow cooker.
2. Cook on low for 3 hours, or until the rice is cooked.
3. Serve hot with topping ingredients

Spicy Brown Rice Burrito Bowl with Cream Cheese

Ingredients:
- 5 Serrano, diced
- 1 red onion, diced
- 1 mild red chili, finely chopped
- 1/2 cup vegan burger (Brand: Beyond Meat Beyond Burger), crumbled
- 1 cup uncooked brown rice
- 1 ½ cups chopped tomatoes
- 1/2 cup water
- 4 tbsp. vegan cream cheese, sliced thinly
- 1 tsp. herbs de Provence
- Sea salt
- Black pepper

Toppings:
- fresh coriander (cilantro), chopped spring onions, sliced avocado, guacamole, etc.

Directions:
1. Combine all the burrito bowl ingredients (not toppings) in a slow cooker.
2. Cook on low for 3 hours, or until the rice is cooked.
3. Serve hot with topping ingredients

Black Rice with Pesto and Anaheim Peppers

Ingredients:
- 1 Anaheim pepper, diced
- 1 red onion, diced
- 1 mild red chili, finely chopped
- 1 1/2 cup fava beans, drained
- 1 cup uncooked black rice
- 1 1/2 cup chopped tomatoes
- 1/2 cup water 4 tbsp. pesto
- 1 tsp. Italian seasoning
- Sea salt
- Black pepper

Toppings:
- fresh coriander (cilantro), chopped spring onions, sliced avocado, guacamole, etc.

Directions:
1. Combine all the burrito bowl ingredients (not toppings) in a slow cooker.
2. Cook on low for 3 hours, or until the rice is cooked.
3. Serve hot with topping ingredients

Brown Rice and Black Beans with Capers

Ingredients:
- 5 jalapeno peppers, diced
- 1 red onion, diced
- 1 mild red chili, finely chopped
- 1 ½ cups black beans, drained
- 1 cup uncooked brown rice
- 1 ½ cups chopped tomatoes
- 1/2 cup water
- 4 tbsp. cream cheese, sliced thinly
- 1/4 cup capers, drained
- Sea salt
- Black pepper

Toppings:
- fresh coriander (cilantro), chopped spring onions, sliced avocado, guacamole, etc.

Directions:
1. Combine all the burrito bowl ingredients (not toppings) in a slow cooker.
2. Cook on low for 3 hours, or until the rice is cooked.
3. Serve hot with topping ingredients

Black Rice with Vegan Chorizo & Olives

Ingredients:

- 1 ancho chili, diced
- 1 red onion, diced
- 1 mild red chili, finely chopped
- 1/4cup capers, drained
- 1/4cup olives, drained
- 1 cup uncooked black rice
- 1/2 cup vegan burger (Brand: Beyond Meat Beyond Burger), crumbled (optional)
- 1/2 cup vegan Chorizo (Soyrizo), crumbled (optional)
- 1 1/2 cup chopped tomatoes
- 1/2 cup water
- 1 tbsp chipotle hot sauce (or other favorite hot sauce)
- 1 tsp smoked paprika
- 1/2 tsp ground cumin
- Sea salt
- Black pepper

Toppings:

- fresh coriander (cilantro), chopped spring onions, sliced avocado, guacamole, etc.

Directions:

1. Combine all the burrito bowl ingredients (not toppings) in a slow cooker.

2. Cook on low for 3 hours, or until the rice is cooked.
3. Serve hot with topping ingredients

Spicy Vegan Chorizo Chili

Ingredients:

- 1 red onion, chopped
- 1 white onion, chopped
- 8 garlic cloves, minced
- 1 tsp. shallot, minced
- 1 15 oz can diced tomatoes
- 4 cups vegetable broth
- 1 can water (I use the can of diced tomatoes to grab all the leftover flavor)
- 8 oz. dried white beans
- 1/2 cup vegan Chorizo (Soyrizo), crumbled
- 2 tablespoons annatto seeds
- 2 teaspoons cumin
- 1 tsp. cayenne pepper
- 1/2 cup uncooked quinoa
- 1/4 teaspoon sea salt

Directions:

1. Put all of the ingredients into a slow cooker.
2. Cook on low for 8 hours or high for 4 hours.
3. Serve with toppings such as shredded vegan cheese, avocado, green onion and cilantro.

Mung Bean and Meatball Chili

Ingredients:

- 2 red onion, chopped
- 7 garlic cloves, minced
- 8 jalapeno peppers, minced
- 1 tbsp. lemon juice
- 4 cups vegetable broth
- 1 can water (I use the can of diced tomatoes to grab all the leftover flavor)
- 8 oz. dried mung beans
- 1/2 cup meatless meatballs, crumbled
- 2 tablespoons garlic, minced
- 2 teaspoons chili powder
- 1 tablespoon Thai chili garlic paste
- 1/2 cup uncooked black rice
- 1/4 teaspoon sea salt

Directions:

1. Put all of the ingredients into a slow cooker.
2. Cook on low for 8 hours or high for 4 hours.
3. Serve with toppings such as shredded vegan cheese, avocado, green onion and cilantro.

Vegan Burger with White and Black Beans

Ingredients:

- 1 red onion, chopped
- 1 white onion, chopped
- 8 garlic cloves, minced
- 1 tsp. shallot, minced
- 1 15 oz can diced tomatoes
- 4 cups vegetable broth
- 1 can water (I use the can of diced tomatoes to grab all the leftover flavor)
- 8 oz. dried white beans
- 1/2 cup vegan burger (Brand: Beyond Meat Beyond Burger), crumbled
- 2 tablespoons annatto seeds
- 2 teaspoons cumin
- 1 tsp. cayenne pepper
- 1/2 cup uncooked brown rice
- 1/4 teaspoon sea salt

Directions:

1. Put all of the ingredients into a slow cooker.
2. Cook on low for 8 hours or high for 4 hours.
3. Serve with toppings such as shredded vegan cheese, avocado, green onion and cilantro.

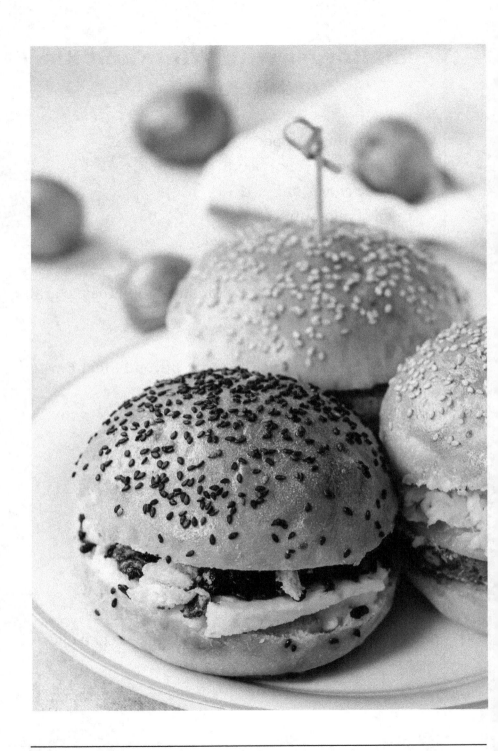

Slow Cooked Lima Beans in Pesto Sauce

Ingredients:
- 1 red onion, chopped
- 2 red onions
- 7 garlic cloves
- 1 ancho chili, minced
- 1 tbsp. lime juice
- 4 cups vegetable broth
- 1 can water (I use the can of diced tomatoes to grab all the leftover flavor)
- 8 oz. dried kidney
- 1 15 oz can Lima Beans
- 3 tablespoons pesto sauce
- 1 teaspoons dried basil, coarsely chopped
- 1 tsp. dried Italian seasoning
- 1/2 cup uncooked rice
- 1/4 teaspoon sea salt

Directions:
1. Put all of the ingredients into a slow cooker.
2. Cook on low for 8 hours or high for 4 hours.
3. Serve with toppings such as shredded vegan cheese, avocado, green onion and cilantro.

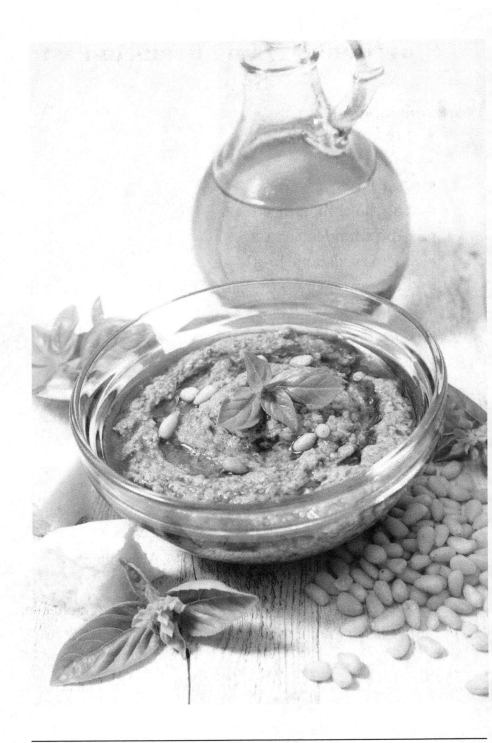

Thai Black Beans Button Mushrooms and Black Rice

Ingredients:

- 1 red onion, chopped
- 1 yellow onion, chopped
- 8 garlic cloves, minced
- 1 tsp. shallot, minced
- 1 15 oz can diced tomatoes
- 1 15 oz can button mushrooms
- 4 cups vegetable broth
- 1 can water (I use the can of diced tomatoes to grab all the leftover flavor)
- 8 oz. dried mung beans
- 1 15 oz can Black Beans
- 2 tablespoons garlic, minced
- 2 teaspoons chili powder
- 1 tablespoon Thai chili garlic paste
- 1/2 cup uncooked black rice
- 1/4 teaspoon sea salt

Directions:

1. Put all of the ingredients into a slow cooker.
2. Cook on low for 8 hours or high for 4 hours.
3. Serve with toppings such as shredded vegan cheese, avocado, green onion and cilantro.

French Lentils & Black Bean With Red Rice

Ingredients:
- 2 red onion, chopped
- 7 garlic cloves, minced
- 1 tsp. scallions, minced
- 1 tbsp. lemon juice
- 1 15 oz can diced tomatoes
- 4 cups vegetable broth
- 1 can water (I use the can of diced tomatoes to grab all the leftover flavor)
- 8 oz. dried lentils
- 1 15 oz can Black Beans
- 2 tablespoons garlic powder
- 2 teaspoons onion powder
- 1 tablespoon herbs de Provence
- 1/2 cup uncooked red rice
- 1/4 teaspoon sea salt

Directions:
1. Put all of the ingredients into a slow cooker.
2. Cook on low for 8 hours or high for 4 hours.
3. Serve with toppings such as shredded vegan cheese, avocado, green onion and cilantro.

Thai Spicy Black Rice and Mung Beans

Ingredients:
- 1 red onion, chopped
- 6 garlic cloves, minced
- 1 celery stalk, chopped
- 2 bell peppers, chopped
- 1 15 oz can diced tomatoes
- 4 cups vegetable broth
- 1 can water (I use the can of diced tomatoes to grab all the leftover flavor)
- 8 oz. dried mung beans
- 1 15 oz can Black Beans
- 2 tablespoons garlic, minced
- 2 teaspoons chili powder
- 1 tablespoon Thai chili garlic paste
- 1/2 cup uncooked black rice
- 1/4 teaspoon sea salt

Directions:
1. Put all of the ingredients into a slow cooker.
2. Cook on low for 8 hours or high for 4 hours.
3. Serve with toppings such as shredded vegan cheese, avocado, green onion and cilantro.

Slow Cooked Tomatoes Rice and Vegan Chorizo

Ingredients:

- 1 red onion, chopped
- 6 garlic cloves, minced
- 1 celery stalk, chopped
- 2 bell peppers, chopped
- 1 15 oz can diced tomatoes
- 4 cups vegetable broth
- 1 can water (I use the can of diced tomatoes to grab all the leftover flavor)
- 1/2 cup vegan Chorizo (Soyrizo), crumbled
- 2 tablespoons annatto seeds
- 2 teaspoons cumin
- 1 tsp. cayenne pepper
- 1/2 cup uncooked brown rice
- 1/4 teaspoon sea salt

Directions:

1. Put all of the ingredients into a slow cooker.
2. Cook on low for 8 hours or high for 4 hours.
3. Serve with toppings such as shredded vegan cheese, avocado, green onion and cilantro.

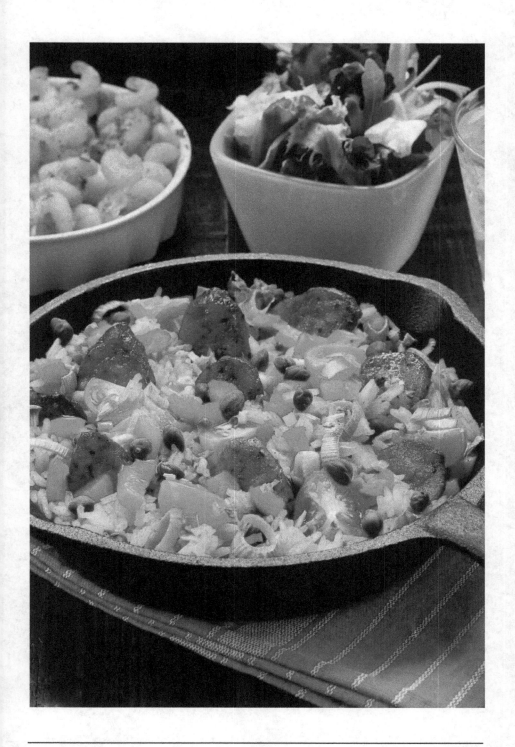

Black Beans and Kidney Beans

Ingredients:

- 2 red onions
- 7 garlic cloves
- 1 ancho chili, minced
- 1 tbsp. lime juice
- 4 cups vegetable broth
- 1 can water (I use the can of diced tomatoes to grab all the leftover flavor)
- 8 oz. dried kidney beans
- 1/2 cup vegan Italian sausage, crumbled
- 3 tablespoons pesto sauce
- 1 teaspoons dried basil, coarsely chopped
- 1 tsp. dried Italian seasoning
- 1/2 cup uncooked rice
- 1/4 teaspoon sea salt

Directions:

1. Put all of the ingredients into a slow cooker.
2. Cook on low for 8 hours or high for 4 hours.
3. Serve with toppings such as shredded vegan cheese, avocado, green onion and cilantro.

Smoky Quinoa and Meatless Meatballs

Ingredients:
- 1 red onion, chopped
- 1 white onion, chopped
- 8 garlic cloves, minced
- 1 tsp. shallot, minced
- 1 15 oz can diced tomatoes
- 4 cups vegetable broth
- 1 can water (I use the can of diced tomatoes to grab all the leftover flavor)
- 1/2 cup meatless meatballs, crumbled
- 2 tablespoons chili powder
- 2 teaspoons cumin
- 1 tablespoon oregano
- 1/2 cup uncooked quinoa
- 1/4 teaspoon sea salt

Directions:
1. Put all of the ingredients into a slow cooker.
2. Cook on low for 8 hours or high for 4 hours.
3. Serve with toppings such as shredded vegan cheese, avocado, green onion and cilantro.

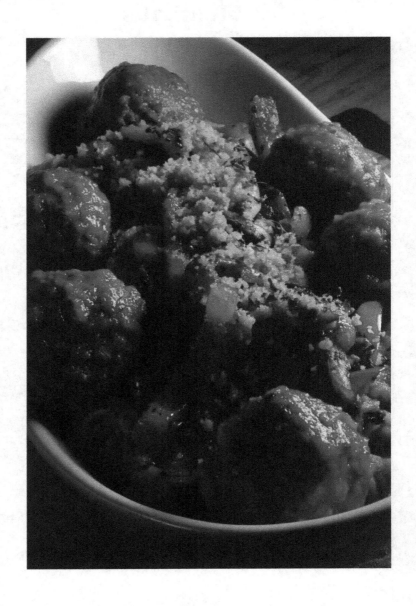

Black Rice with Enoki Mushrooms

Ingredients:

- 2 red onion, chopped
- 7 garlic cloves, minced
- 8 jalapeno peppers, minced
- 1 tbsp. lemon juice
- 4 cups vegetable broth
- 1 can water (I use the can of diced tomatoes to grab all the leftover flavor)
- 8 oz. dried mung beans
- 1 15 oz can enoki mushrooms
- 2 tablespoons garlic, minced
- 2 teaspoons chili powder
- 1 tablespoon Thai chili garlic paste
- 1/2 cup uncooked black rice
- 1/4 teaspoon sea salt

Directions:

1. Put all of the ingredients into a slow cooker.
2. Cook on low for 8 hours or high for 4 hours.
3. Serve with toppings such as shredded vegan cheese, avocado, green onion and cilantro.

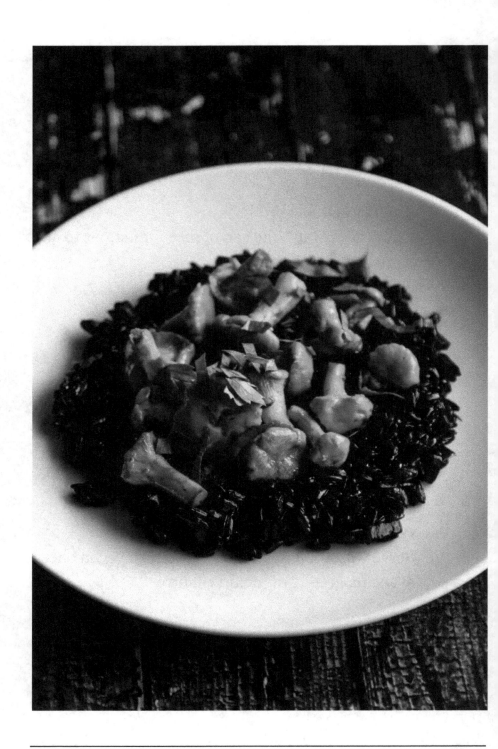

Red Rice with Enoki Mushrooms and Tomatoes

Ingredients:

- 1 red onion, chopped
- 6 garlic cloves, minced
- 1 celery stalk, chopped
- 2 bell peppers, chopped
- 1 15 oz can diced tomatoes
- 4 cups vegetable broth
- 1 can water (I use the can of diced tomatoes to grab all the leftover flavor)
- 8 oz. dried lentils
- 1 15 oz can enoki mushrooms
- 2 tablespoons garlic powder
- 2 teaspoons onion powder
- 1 tablespoon herbs de Provence
- 1/2 cup uncooked red rice
- 1/4 teaspoon sea salt

Directions:

1. Put all of the ingredients into a slow cooker.
2. Cook on low for 8 hours or high for 4 hours.
3. Serve with toppings such as shredded vegan cheese, avocado, green onion and cilantro.

Brown Rice with Crimini Mushrooms and Jalapeno Pepper

Ingredients:

- 2 red onion, chopped
- 7 garlic cloves, minced
- 8 jalapeno peppers, minced
- 1 tbsp. lemon juice
- 4 cups vegetable broth
- 1 can water (I use the can of diced tomatoes to grab all the leftover flavor)
- 1 15 oz can crimini mushrooms
- 2 tablespoons annatto seeds
- 2 teaspoons cumin
- 1 tsp. cayenne pepper
- 1/2 cup uncooked brown rice
- 1/4 teaspoon sea salt

Directions:

1. Put all of the ingredients into a slow cooker.
2. Cook on low for 8 hours or high for 4 hours.
3. Serve with toppings such as shredded vegan cheese, avocado, green onion and cilantro.

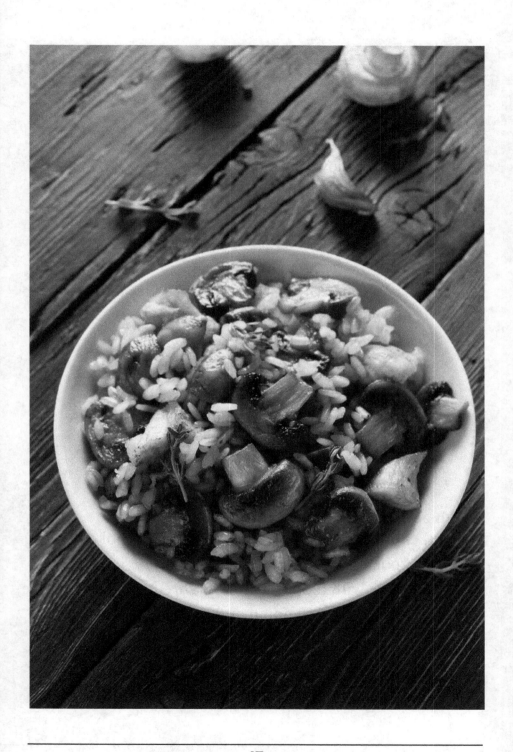

Rice with Pesto Sauce and Button Mushrooms

Ingredients:

- 1 red onion, chopped
- 6 garlic cloves, minced
- 1 celery stalk, chopped
- 2 bell peppers, chopped
- 1 15 oz can diced tomatoes
- 4 cups vegetable broth
- 1 can water (I use the can of diced tomatoes to grab all the leftover flavor)
- 1 15 oz can button mushrooms
- 3 tablespoons pesto sauce
- 1 teaspoons dried basil, coarsely chopped
- 1 tsp. dried Italian seasoning
- 1/2 cup uncooked rice
- 1/4 teaspoon sea salt

Directions:

1. Put all of the ingredients into a slow cooker.
2. Cook on low for 8 hours or high for 4 hours.
3. Serve with toppings such as shredded vegan cheese, avocado, green onion and cilantro.

Red Rice with Crimini and Button Mushrooms

Ingredients:

- 2 red onion, chopped
- 7 garlic cloves, minced
- 1 tsp. scallions, minced
- 1 tbsp. lemon juice
- 4 cups vegetable broth
- 1 can water (I use the can of diced tomatoes to grab all the leftover flavor)
- 1 cup crimini mushrooms
- 1 cup button mushrooms
- 2 tablespoons garlic powder
- 2 teaspoons onion powder
- 1 tablespoon herbs de Provence
- 1/2 cup uncooked red rice
- 1/4 teaspoon sea salt

Directions:

1. Put all of the ingredients into a slow cooker.
2. Cook on low for 8 hours or high for 4 hours.
3. Serve with toppings such as shredded vegan cheese, avocado, green onion and cilantro.

Veggie Pie

Ingredients:

- 7 cups vegetables chopped into bite sized pieces as needed (I used: brussel sprouts, frozen corn kernels, frozen peas, diced potatoes, baby carrots, and pre-sliced mushrooms)
- 1/2 cup diced red onion
- 4 cloves minced garlic
- 5-6 sprigs fresh thyme leaves removed
- 1/4 cup flour
- 2 cups chicken stock
- 1/4 cup cornstarch
- 1/4 cup heavy cream
- salt and pepper to taste
- 1 frozen puff pastry sheet thawed
- 2 tablespoons olive oil

Directions:

1. Put the 7 cups of vegetables as needed to your slow cooker together with the onion and garlic.
2. Combine with the flour to coat well.
3. Add the broth until well combined with the flour.
4. Cover and cook on high heat for 3 and a half hours or low heat for 6 and a half hours.
5. Combine cornstarch with 1/4 cup water until smooth and add this to the slow cooker.
6. Add the coconut cream, cover, and return the slow cooker.

7. Cook on high for 15 minutes or until mixture thickens.
8. Transfer to a baking dish and top with the thawed puff pastry sheet.
9. Brush the olive oil over the top of the pastry.
10. Bake at 400 degrees F for about 10 minutes or until pastry turns golden brown.

Soy Bean and Bell Pepper Soup

Ingredients:

- 1 pound dry soy beans
- 4 cups vegetable stock
- 1 yellow onion, finely chopped
- 1 green bell pepper, finely chopped
- 2 jalapeños, seeds removed and finely chopped
- 1 cup salsa or diced tomatoes
- 4 teaspoons minced garlic, about 4 cloves
- 1 heaping tablespoon chili powder
- 2 teaspoons ground cumin
- 2 teaspoons sea salt
- 1 teaspoon ground pepper
- 1/2 teaspoon ground cayenne pepper (decrease or omit for a milder soup)
- 1/2 teaspoon smoked paprika Avocado and cilantro for topping, if desired

Directions:

1. Completely submerge the beans in water overnight and make sure there's an inch of water over the beans.
2. Drain the beans and rinse.
3. Put the beans, broth, onion, pepper, jalapeños, salsa, garlic, chili powder, cumin, salt, pepper, cayenne, and paprika in a slow cooker.
4. Stir and combine thoroughly.
5. Cook on high heat for 6 hours, until beans are tender.

6. Blend half of the soup until smooth and bring it back to the pot.
7. Top with avocado and cilantro.

Masala Brown ,Green and Pardina Lentils

Ingredients:

- 1 red onion, chopped
- 5 cloves garlic, minced
- 1 tablespoon minced fresh ginger, or 1 teaspoon ground ginger powder
- 2¼ cups brown, green or pardina lentils
- 4 cups vegetable broth
- 1 15-ounce can diced
- San Marzano tomatoes, with their juices
- ¼ cup tomato paste
- 2 teaspoons tamarind paste (optional, adds a hint of tartness)
- 1 teaspoon honey
- ¾ teaspoon sea salt
- 1½ teaspoon garam masala
- A few shakes black pepper
- 1 cup light coconut milk

Side dish:

- Rice, quinoa, or another whole grain and fresh herbs

Directions:

1. Put everything except for the coconut milk and side dish ingredients in the slow cooker.

2. Combine thoroughly and cook on high for 3 and a half hours or on low for 6 hours. In the last hour, check if more liquid needs to be added..
3. When the lentils become more tender, add the coconut milk. Add this to the rice, quinoa and fresh herbs.

Swiss Chard and White Bean Stew

Ingredients:

- 2 pounds white beans (sorted and rinsed)
- 2 large carrots, peeled and diced
- 3 large celery stalks, diced
- 1 red onion, diced
- 6 cloves garlic, minced or chopped
- 1 bay leaf
- 1 tsp. each: dried rosemary, thyme, oregano
- 11 cups water
- 2 Tbsp. salt
- Ground black pepper, to taste
- 1 large can (28 ounces) diced tomatoes
- 5-6 cups chopped Swiss chard & kale Rice, polenta, or bread for serving

Directions:

1. Combine beans, carrots, celery, onions, garlic, bay leaf and dried herbs.
2. Add the water.
3. Cook on high heat for 3 ½ hours, or low heat for 9 hours.
4. Remove the lid from the slow cooker and season with salt and pepper.
5. Add diced tomatoes.
6. Cook for another 1 hour and 15 min. or until beans get very soft.
7. Garnish with the chopped greens.
8. Serve with cooked rice, polenta, or with bread.

Faro and Kidney Bean Chili

Ingredients:

- 1 cup uncooked farro
- 1 medium red or yellow onion, peeled and diced
- 8 cloves of garlic, minced
- 1 chipotle chili in adobo sauce, chopped
- 2 (15 ounce) vans dark red kidney beans, rinsed and drained

  (**see below for substitution ideas)
- 2 (15 ounce) cans tomato sauce
- 2 (14 ounce) cans diced tomatoes
- 1 (15 ounce) can light red kidney beans, rinsed and drained
- 1 (4 ounce) can chopped red chilies
- 4 cups vegetable broth
- 1 cup beer (or you can just add extra vegetable broth)
- 2 Tablespoons chili powder
- 1 Tablespoon ground cumin
- 1 teaspoon sea salt
- 1 teaspoon honey
- 1/2 teaspoon black pepper

Directions:

1. Combine all of the ingredients in a slow cooker and stir thoroughly.
2. Cook on high for 3 ½ hours or on low heat for 7 hours until the beans are soft.

---

3. Taste, and add more salt and pepper if necessary.
4. Garnish with toppings.
5. Refrigerate for 3 days or freeze for 3 months.

Avocado Lima Beans and Tomato Bowl

Ingredients:
- 1/2 cup Lima Beans, warmed
- 1 teaspoon extra-virgin olive oil
- 1/2 cup Roma tomatoes
- 1/4 cup fresh corn kernels (from 1 ear)
- 1/2 medium-sized ripe avocado, thinly sliced
- 1 medium radish, very thinly sliced
- 2 tablespoons fresh cilantro leaves
- 1/4 teaspoon sea salt
- 1/8 teaspoon black pepper

Directions:
1. Heat the skillet over medium high heat.
2. Add oil to the pan.
3. Add tomatoes to the oil and cook until tender but charred for about 3 minutes.
4. Set the tomatoes beside the beans in a large bowl.
5. Cook the corn and cook for 2 ½ min.
6. Place the corn next to the tomatoes.
7. Add avocado, radish, and cilantro.
8. Season with salt and pepper.

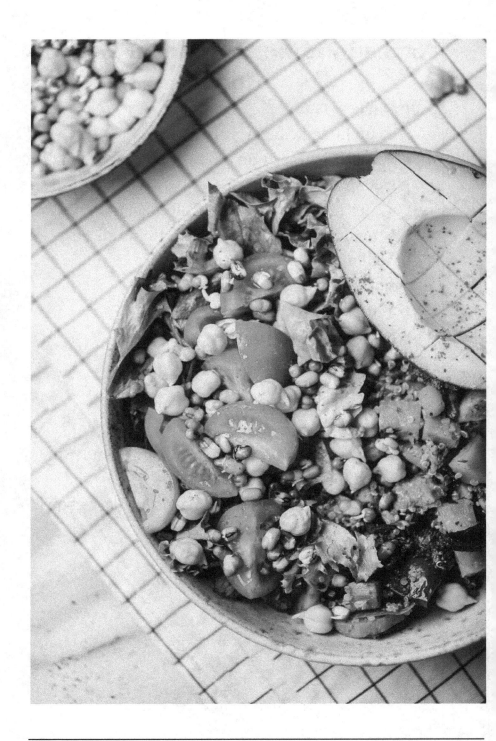

Brussels Tempeh with Soy Dressing

Ingredients:

- 2 tablespoons sesame oil, divided
- 4 ounces tempeh, thinly sliced
- 4 teaspoons soy sauce
- 2 teaspoons sherry vinegar
- 1/8 teaspoon sea salt
- 2 tablespoons chopped fresh cilantro, divided
- 2 beetroots, peeled and sliced lengthwise
- Thin jalapeno chili slices
- 2 tablespoons chopped unsalted peanuts, toasted
- 2 lime wedges

Directions:

1. Heat a pan over medium-high.
2. Heat 1 tablespoon of the oil in the pan.
3. Add tempeh and cook until very crisp and browned, about 2 minutes per side.
4. Transfer to a plate.
5. Combine the soy sauce, vinegar, salt, 1 tablespoon of the cilantro, and the remaining sesame oil in a bowl.
6. Add the Brussels sprouts, and mix to coat.
7. Divide between 2 bowls.
8. Sprinkle with jalapeno chili slices and peanuts, and top with the tempeh slices.
9. Pour the remaining dressing, and top with the remaining cilantro.
10. Serve with lime wedges.

Quinoa with Pesto Cream

Ingredients:

- Pesto Cream
- 2 large bunches basil (about 2 cups lightly packed leaves)
- 1/4 cup extra virgin olive oil
- 1/4 cup cream
- 1 garlic clove
- 1 tsp pecorino romano cheese
- Sea salt and pepper to taste

Quinoa Filling:

- 1 tbsp extra virgin olive oil
- 1 medium red onion, diced
- 10 oz fresh spinach
- 3 garlic cloves
- 1/2 tsp Italian seasoning
- 3 cups cooked quinoa
- 6 Tbsp vegan pesto
- Sea salt Black pepper to taste

Tomatoes:

- 6 large tomatoes, (seeds and cores scooped out)
- 2 Tbsp extra virgin olive oil
- Sea salt and pepper to taste
- fresh basil
- Preheat your oven to 400 degrees F.

Directions:

1. Combine all of the pesto ingredients in a blender and blend until smooth.
2. In a pan, sauté the onion in olive oil for 7 minutes or until translucent.
3. Add the spinach and garlic cloves and cook for 2 more minutes .
4. Add the cooked quinoa, pesto sauce, Italian seasonings, salt, and pepper.
5. Cut the top off each tomato.
6. Scoop out all the seeds.
7. Drizzle olive oil in a baking pan and spread it around.
8. Place the tomatoes in the baking pan and drizzle with a tbsp of oil over the top of the tomatoes.
9. Season with salt & pepper.
10. Ladle the pesto quinoa filling into each of the tomatoes and put the tops back on.
11. Roast for 30 minutes.
12. Garnish with basil.

Southeast Asian Fried Rice

Ingredients:

- 1 cup raw short grain rice
- 1 red onion, chopped
- 6 cloves of garlic, chopped
- 1 tablespoon olive oil
- 2 carrots, cut into thin sticks
- 1/2 green bell pepper, cut into thin sticks
- 1/2 cup frozen peas
- 1/2 cup cashews
- 1 tablespoon soy sauce
- 1 tablespoon red curry powder
- 1 cup pineapple, cut into small pieces
- 2 green onions, cut into rings
- Sea salt, to taste
- black pepper, to taste
- red pepper flakes
- fresh cilantro (optional)

Directions:

1. Cook the rice according to package instructions.
2. Cook the peas for 7 minutes.
3. Heat the oil in a pan and cook the onion for about 3 minutes.
4. Add the garlic, the carrots, and the bell pepper and cook for 3 minutes.

5. Add the rice and season with curry powder and the soy sauce.
6. Add the pineapple, the peas, the green onion, and cashews.
7. Sprinkle with salt, black pepper, and if using red pepper flakes.

Curried Lima Beans

Ingredients:
- 2 Tbsp extra virgin olive oil
- 1 medium red onion , diced
- 4 cloves garlic , minced
- 2 15 oz can lima beans, drained
- 1 20 oz can tomato sauce
- 1 cup water
- 1 Tbsp red curry powder
- 1/2 bunch fresh cilantro , rinsed and stems removed and coarsely chopped

Directions:
1. Stir fry the onion and garlic in a pan with olive oil over medium heat until softened (takes about 4 minutes).
2. Drain the beans and add to the pan.
3. Add the tomato sauce, water and curry powder.
4. Stir everything until it is well-mixed.
5. Simmer over medium heat.
6. Add cilantro to the pot.
7. Stir and simmer until the sauce has a thick consistency.

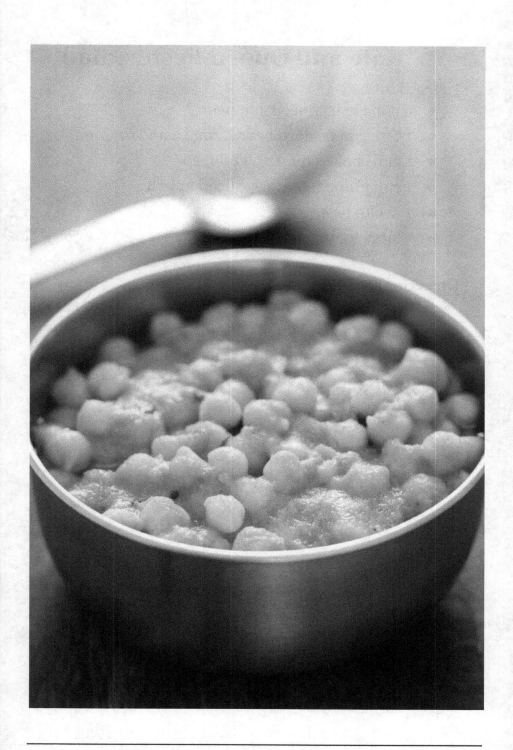

Kale and Quorn Pesto Salad

Ingredients:

- 6 cups kale, finely chopped
- 15 oz. can borlotti beans, rinsed and drained
- 1 cup cooked quorn*, chopped
- 1 cup grape tomatoes, sliced in half
- 1/2 cup pesto
- 1 large lemon, cut into wedges

Directions:

1. Combine all of the ingredients in a bowl except for the pesto and lemon.
2. Add the pesto and toss until coated.

Vegetarian Tofu Wrap

Ingredients:

- 1/2 red cabbage, shredded
- 4 heaped tbsp dairy-free yogurt
- 3 tbsp mint sauce
- 3 x 7 ounce packs tofu, each cut into 15 cubes
- 2 tbsp tandoori curry paste
- 2 tbsp extra virgin olive oil
- 2 red onions, sliced
- 2 large garlic cloves, sliced
- 8 chapatis 2 limes, cut into quarters

Directions:

1. Combine the cabbage, dairy-free yogurt and mint sauce in a bowl.
2. Season with salt and pepper and set aside.
3. Combine the tofu ,tandoori paste and 1 tbsp of the oil.
4. Heat oil on a pan and cook the tofu in batches until golden.
5. Take the tofu off the pan.
6. Add the remaining oil, stir fry the onions and garlic, and cook for 9 mins .
7. Return the tofu to the pan.
8. Add more salt.
9. To Assemble Warm the chapattis following package instructions.
10. Top each one with cabbage, tofu and a squeeze of lime juice.

Vegetarian Navy Bean Chili

Ingredients:
- 2 tbsp extra virgin olive oil
- 6 garlic cloves, finely chopped
- 2 large red onions, chopped
- 3 tbsp sweet pimenton or mild chili powder
- 3 tbsp ground cumin
- Sea salt, to taste
- 3 tbsp cider vinegar
- 2 tbsp honey
- 2 (14 oz.) cans chopped tomatoes
- 2 (14 oz.) cans navy beans, rinsed and drained

For garnishing:
- crumbled vegan cheese, chopped spring onions, sliced radishes, avocado chunks, soured cream

Directions:
1. Heat the olive oil and fry the garlic and onions until softened.
2. Stir in the pimenton and cumin, cook for 3 mins.
3. Add the vinegar, honey, tomatoes and sea salt.
4. Cook for 10 more mins.
5. Add the beans and cook for another 10 mins.
6. Serve with rice and sprinkle with the garnishing ingredients.

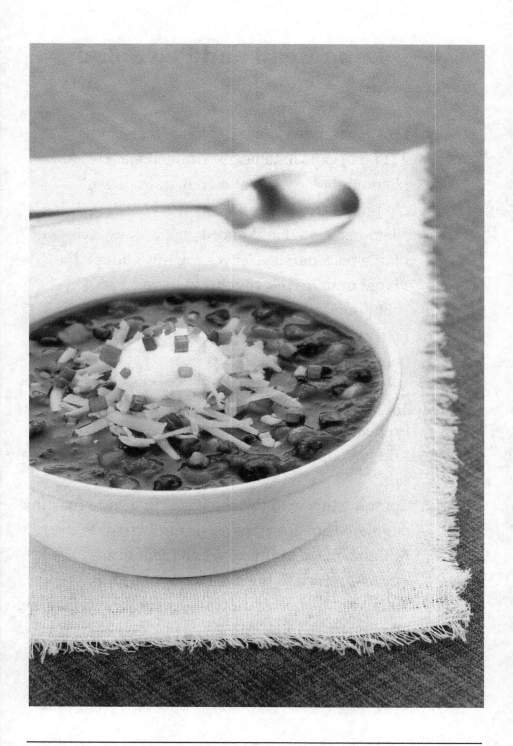

Lima Bean and Pea Salad

Ingredients:
- 1/2 cup extra virgin olive oil
- 1 tbsp garam masala
- 2 (14 oz.) cans lima beans, drained and rinsed
- 1/2 pound ready-to-eat mixed grain pouch
- 1/2 pound frozen peas
- 2 lemons, zested and juiced
- 1 large pack parsley, leaves roughly chopped
- 1 large mint leaves, roughly chopped
- Half pound radishes, roughly chopped
- 1 cucumber, chopped
- pomegranate seeds, to serve

Directions:
1. Preheat your oven to 392 degrees F.
2. Add 1/4 cup oil with the garam masala and add some salt.
3. Combine this with the chickpeas in a large roasting pan then cook for 15 mins. or until crisp.
4. Add the mixed grains, peas and lemon zest.
5. Stir and return to the oven for about 10 mins.
6. Toss with the herbs, radishes, cucumber, remaining oil and lemon juice.
7. Season with more salt and garnish with the pomegranate seeds.

Broccoli & Basmati Rice Pilaf

Ingredients:
- 1 tbsp olive oil
- 2 large red onions, sliced
- 1 tbsp curry paste of your choice
- 1/2 pound basmati rice
- 3/4 pound broccoli florets
- 1 pound chickpeas, rinsed and drained
- 2 cups vegetable stock
- 1/8 cup toasted flaked almonds handful chopped coriander

Directions:
1. Heat the oil in a pan and cook the onions over medium heat for 5 mins until it starts to brown.
2. Add the curry paste and cook for 1 min.
3. Add in the rice, broccoli and chickpeas.
4. Combine all of this to coat.
5. Add in the stock and combine thoroughly.
6. Cover and simmer for 12 ½ mins or until the rice and broccoli become tender and all the liquid has been reduced.
7. Add the almonds and coriander.

Avocado and Lima Bean Salad Sandwich

Ingredients:

- 1 15-oz. can lima beans, rinsed, drained, and skinned
- 1 large, ripe avocado
- 1/4 cup chopped fresh cilantro
- 2 Tbsp. chopped green onions
- Juice of 1 lime
- Sea salt and pepper, to taste
- Bread of your choice

Directions:

1. Lettuce Tomato Mash the lima beans and avocado with a fork.
2. Add cilantro , green onions, and lime juice and stir Season with salt and pepper.
3. Spread on your favorite bread and garnish with lettuce and tomato

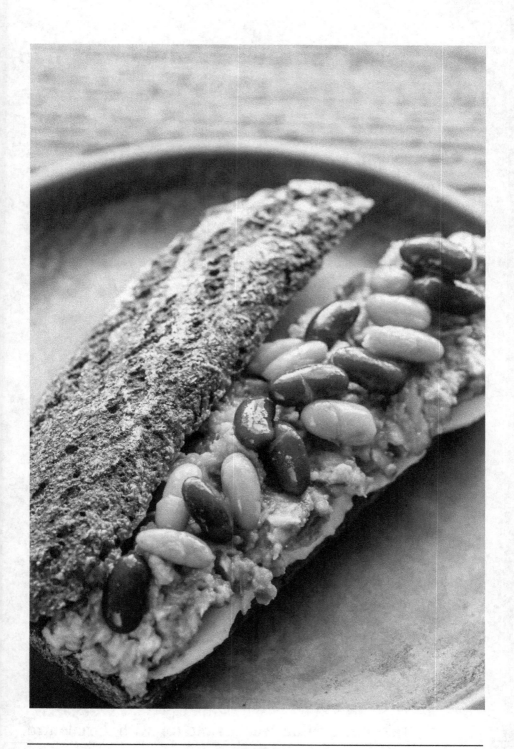

Roasted Cauliflower and Garbanzo Beans

Ingredients:
- cooking spray
- 1 tablespoon extra virgin olive oil
- 3 cloves garlic, minced
- 1/2 teaspoon sea salt
- 1/4 teaspoon ground black pepper
- 3 1/2 cups sliced cauliflower
- 2 1/2 cups grape tomatoes
- 1 (15 ounce) can garbanzo beans, drained
- 1 lime, cut into wedges
- 1 tablespoon chopped fresh cilantro

Directions:
1. Preheat your oven to 450 degrees F. Line a baking sheet with foil and grease with olive oil. Mix the olive oil, garlic, salt, and pepper in a bowl.
2. Add in the cauliflower, tomatoes, and garbanzo beans.
3. Combine until well coated.
4. Spread them out in a single layer on the baking sheet.
5. Add the lime wedges.
6. Roast in the oven until vegetables become caramelized, for about 25 minutes.
7. Take out the lime wedges and top with the cilantro.

Roasted Tomato Broccoli and Chickpeas

Ingredients:
- cooking spray
- 1 tablespoon extra virgin olive oil
- 5 cloves garlic, minced
- 1/2 teaspoon sea salt
- 1/4 teaspoon ground black pepper
- 3 1/2 cups sliced broccoli
- 2 1/2 cups grape tomatoes
- 1/2 tsp. annatto seeds
- 1/2 cup green olives
- 1/2 cup capers
- 1 (15 ounce) can chickpeas, drained
- 1 lime, cut into wedges
- 1 tablespoon chopped fresh cilantro

Directions:
1. Preheat your oven to 450 degrees F.
2. Line a baking sheet with foil and grease with olive oil.
3. Mix the olive oil, garlic, annatto seeds, salt, and pepper in a bowl.
4. Add in the broccoli, capers, olives, tomatoes, and garbanzo beans.
5. Combine until well coated.
6. Spread them out in a single layer on the baking sheet.

---

7. Add the lime wedges.
8. Roast in the oven until vegetables become caramelized, for about 25 minutes.
9. Take out the lime wedges and top with the cilantro.

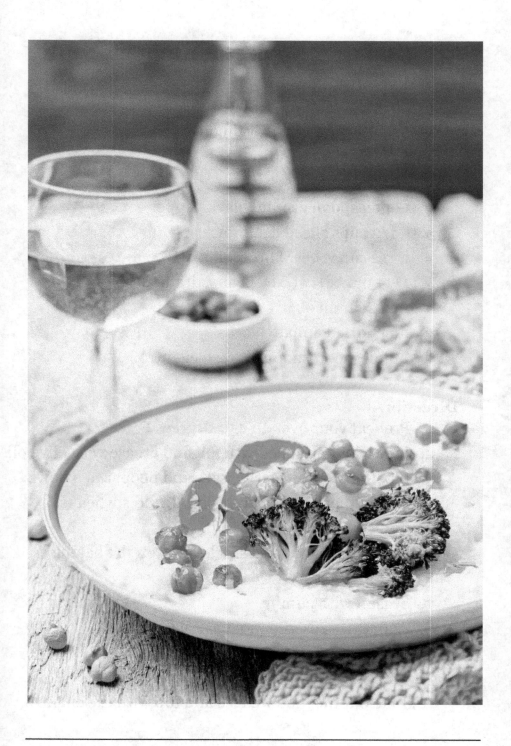

Roasted Soybean and Broccoli

Ingredients:

- cooking spray
- 1 tablespoon extra virgin olive oil
- 3 cloves garlic, minced
- 1/2 teaspoon sea salt
- 1/4 teaspoon ground black pepper
- 3 1/2 cups sliced cauliflower
- 2 1/2 cups cherry broccoli
- 1 (15 ounce) can soy beans, drained
- 1 tsp. cumin
- 1 tsp. dried annatto seeds
- 1 tablespoon chopped fresh cilantro

Directions:

1. Preheat your oven to 450 degrees F.
2. Line a baking sheet with foil and grease with olive oil.
3. Mix the olive oil, garlic, salt, and pepper in a bowl.
4. Add in the cauliflower, broccoli, and soybeans.
5. Combine until well coated.
6. Spread them out in a single layer on the baking sheet.
7. Season with cumin.
8. Annatto seeds and more salt if necessary.
9. Roast in the oven until vegetables become caramelized, for about 25 minutes.
10. Take out the lime wedges and top with the cilantro.

Buttery Roasted Tomatoes and Edamame Beans

Ingredients:
- cooking spray
- 1 tablespoon melted butter
- 8 cloves garlic, minced
- 1/2 teaspoon sea salt
- 1/4 teaspoon Italian seasoning
- 3 1/2 cups sliced cauliflower
- 2 1/2 cups cherry tomatoes
- 1 (15 ounce) can edamame beans, drained
- 1 lime, cut into wedges
- 1/4 cup green olives

Directions:
1. Preheat your oven to 450 degrees F.
2. Line a baking sheet with foil and grease with olive oil.
3. Mix the olive oil, garlic, salt, and Italian seasoning in a bowl.
4. Add in the cauliflower, green olives, tomatoes, and edamame beans.
5. Combine until well coated.
6. Spread them out in a single layer on the baking sheet.
7. Add the lime wedges.
8. Roast in the oven until vegetables become caramelized, for about 25 minutes.

9. Take out the lime wedges and top with the cilantro.

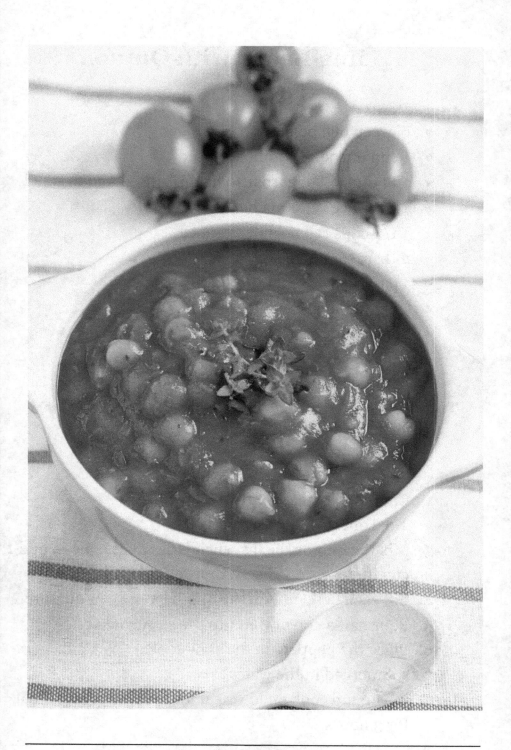

Lima Beans with Quinoa

Ingredients:
- 6 green bell peppers
- 1 cup uncooked quinoa, rinsed
- 1 14 ounce can garbanzo beans, rinsed and drained
- 1 14 ounce can lima beans
- 1 1/2 cups red enchilada sauce
- 2 tbsp. tomato paste
- 1 tsp. basil
- 1 tsp. Italian seasoning
- 1/2 teaspoon garlic powder
- ½ tsp. sea salt
- 1 1/2 cups shredded mozzarella cheese

Toppings:
- cilantro, avocado

Directions:
1. Cut out the stems of the bell pepper.
2. Take out the ribs and the seeds.
3. Mix the quinoa, beans, enchilada sauce, spices, and 1 cup of the vegan cheese thoroughly.
4. Fill each pepper with the quinoa and bean mixture.
5. Pour half a cup of water to the slow cooker.
6. Place the peppers in the slow cooker (partially submerged in the water).
7. Cover and cook on low heat for 6 hours or high heat for 3 hours.

8. Uncover and distribute the remaining vegan cheese over the tops of the peppers, and cover for 4 to 5 minutes to melt the cheese.
9. Top with cilantro & avocado

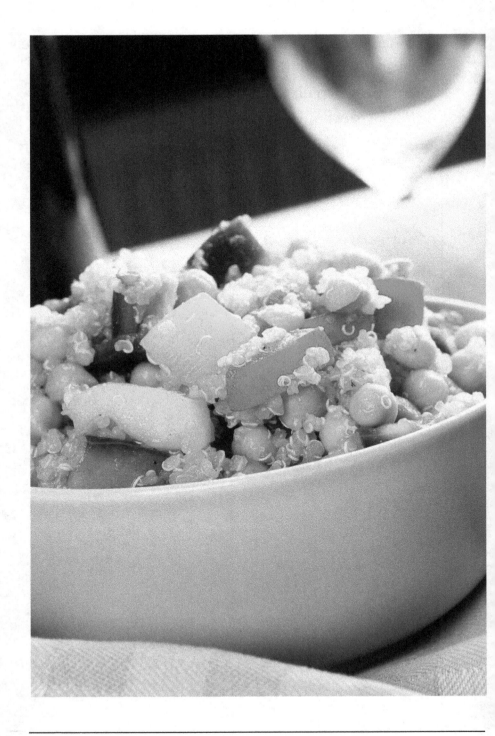

Vegetarian Brown Rice Burrito Bowl

Ingredients:

- 1 red onion, diced or thinly sliced
- 1 green bell pepper (I used yellow), diced
- 1/4 cup gouda cheese, shredded
- 1 mild red chili, finely chopped
- 1 ½ cups black beans, drained
- 1 cup uncooked brown rice
- 1 ½ cups chopped tomatoes
- 1/2 cup water
- 1 tbsp chipotle hot sauce (or other favorite hot sauce)
- 1 tsp smoked paprika
- 1/2 tsp ground cumin
- Sea salt
- Black pepper

Toppings:

- fresh coriander (cilantro), chopped spring onions, sliced avocado, guacamole, etc.

Directions:

1. Combine all the burrito bowl ingredients (not toppings) in a slow cooker.
2. Cook on low for 3 hours, or until the rice is cooked.
3. Serve hot with coriander, spring onions, avocado and guacamole.

Garbanzo Bean Burrito Bowl with Sun-dried Pesto

Ingredients:

- 5 jalapeno peppers, diced
- 1 red onion, diced
- 1 mild red chili, finely chopped
- 1 ½ cups garbanzo beans, drained
- 1 cup uncooked red rice
- 1 ½ cups chopped tomatoes
- ½ cup water
- 4 tbsp. sun-dried tomato pesto
- 1 tsp. Italian seasoning
- Sea salt
- Black pepper

Toppings:

- fresh coriander (cilantro), chopped spring onions, sliced avocado, guacamole, etc.

Directions:

1. Combine all the burrito bowl ingredients (not toppings) in a slow cooker.
2. Cook on low for 3 hours, or until the rice is cooked.
3. Serve hot with topping ingredients

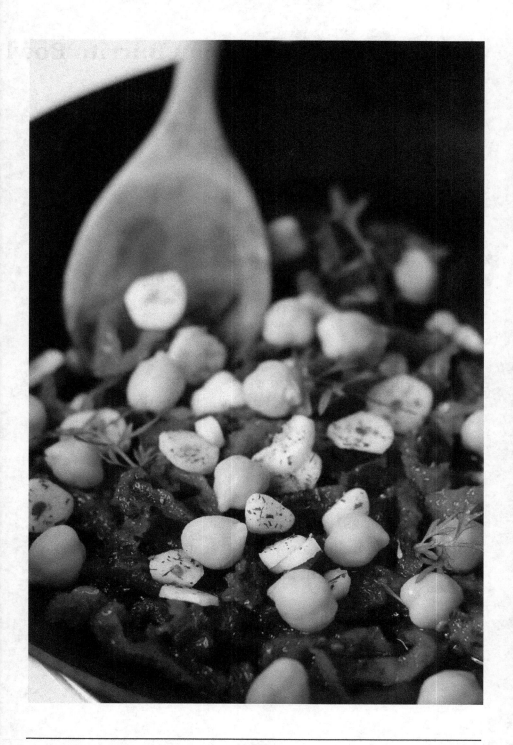

White Bean Vegetarian Burrito Bowl

Ingredients:
- 1 Anaheim pepper, diced
- 1 red onion, diced
- 1 mild red chili, finely chopped
- 1 1/2 cup white beans
- 1 cup uncooked white rice
- 1 1/2 cups chopped tomatoes
- 1/2 cup water
- 4 tbsp. pepper jack cheese, shredded
- 1 tsp. herbs de Provence
- Sea salt
- Black pepper

Toppings:
- fresh coriander (cilantro), chopped spring onions, sliced avocado, guacamole, etc.

Directions:
1. Combine all the burrito bowl ingredients (not toppings) in a slow cooker.
2. Cook on low for 3 hours, or until the rice is cooked.
3. Serve hot with topping ingredients.

Vegetarian Garbanzo Bean Burrito Bowl

Ingredients:

- 1 red onion, diced or thinly sliced
- 1 green bell pepper (I used yellow), diced
- 1 mild red chili, finely chopped
- 1 ½ cups garbanzo beans, drained
- 1 cup uncooked red rice
- 1 ½ cups chopped San Marzano tomatoes
- ½ cup water
- 1 tbsp chipotle hot sauce (or other favorite hot sauce)
- 1 tsp smoked paprika
- 1/2 tsp ground cumin
- Sea salt
- Black pepper

Toppings:

- fresh coriander (cilantro), chopped spring onions, sliced avocado, guacamole, etc.

Directions:

1. Combine all the burrito bowl ingredients (not toppings) in a slow cooker.
2. Cook on low for 3 hours, or until the rice is cooked.
3. Serve hot with topping ingredients

White Bean and Ricotta Cheese Burrito Bowl

Ingredients:

- 1 ancho chili, diced
- 1 red onion, diced
- 1 mild red chili, finely chopped
- 1 1/2 cup white beans
- 1 cup uncooked white rice
- 1 1/2 cups chopped tomatoes
- 1/2 cup water
- 8 tbsp. Ricotta cheese, sliced thinly
- 1 tsp. herbs de Provence
- Sea salt
- Black pepper

Toppings:

- fresh coriander (cilantro), chopped spring onions, sliced avocado, guacamole, etc.

Directions:

1. Combine all the burrito bowl ingredients (not toppings) in a slow cooker.
2. Cook on low for 3 hours, or until the rice is cooked.
3. Serve hot with topping ingredients

Lentils and Sweet Potato Curry

Ingredients:

- 3 large sweet potatoes, diced (about 6 cups)
- 3 cups vegetable stock
- 1 red onion, minced
- 6 cloves garlic, minced
- 2 teaspoon each ground coriander, garam masala, and chili powder
- 1/2 teaspoon sea salt
- 1 1/2 cups uncooked red lentils (masoor dal)
- 1 can coconut milk
- 1 cup water combines the sweet potatoes, vegetable stock, onion, garlic, and spices in a slow cooker.

Directions:

1. Cook on high heat in a slow cooker for 3 hours or until vegetables become soft.
2. Add the lentils and combine.
3. Cook on high for another hour and a half.
4. Add the coconut milk.
5. Add water as needed.

Baked Green Beans and Sweet Potatoes

Ingredients:
- 1 1/2 pounds sweet potatoes, cut into chunks
- 2 tablespoons extra virgin olive oil
- 8 cloves garlic, thinly sliced
- 4 teaspoons dried rosemary
- 4 teaspoons dried thyme
- 2 teaspoons sea salt
- 1 bunch fresh green beans, trimmed and cut into
- 1 inch pieces ground black pepper to taste

Directions:
1. Preheat your oven to 425 degrees F.
2. Combine the potatoes with 1 tbsp. of olive oil, garlic, rosemary, thyme, and 1 tsp. sea salt.
3. Wrap with aluminum foil.
4. Roast for 20 minutes in the oven.
5. Combine the green beans, remaining olive oil, and remaining salt.
6. Cover, and cook for another 15 minutes, until the potatoes are tender.
7. Increase your oven temperature to 450 degrees F .
8. Take out the foil, and cook for 8 minutes, until potatoes are browned.
9. Sprinkle it with pepper.

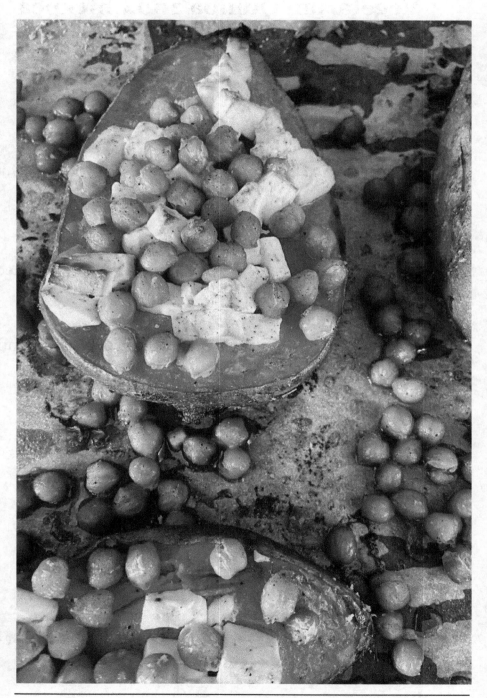

Vegetarian Quinoa and Chickpea Burger

Ingredients:

- 1 1/2 cups cooked quinoa
- 2 tablespoons Dijon mustard
- 1 egg vegan (Brand: Follow Your Heart Egg Vegan), beaten
- 2 cloves garlic, minced
- 2 grinds fresh black pepper
- 1/2 cup chickpea (garbanzo bean) flour, or as needed
- 2 teaspoons olive oil, or as needed
- 2 slices gouda cheese
- Combine the quinoa, mustard, vegan egg, garlic, and black pepper together in a bowl; add enough chickpea flour to make 2 patties.

Directions:

1. Heat oil in a pan over medium heat.
2. Cook patties in oil until browned for around 4 minutes per side.
3. Add a vegan cheese slice to each patty and warm until the cheese melts, about 2 and a half minutes.

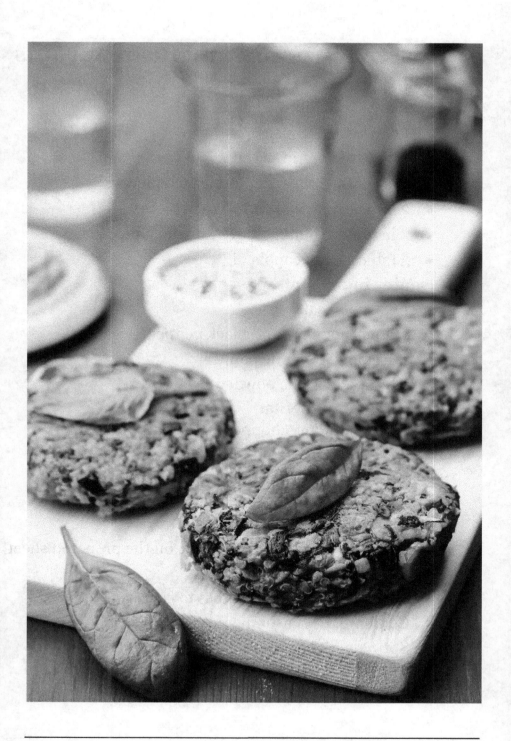

Roasted Broccoli and Bean Sprouts

Ingredients:
- 1 large broccoli, sliced
- 1 cup bean sprouts
- 1 large red onion, diced
- 3 large Rutabaga, cut into 1 inch pieces
- 2 large carrots, cut into 1 inch pieces
- 3 medium potatoes, cut into 1-inch pieces
- 3 tablespoons canola oil

Seasoning ingredients:
- 1 teaspoon salt
- 1/2 teaspoon ground black pepper
- 1 teaspoon cayenne pepper
- 2 teaspoon garlic powder

Garnishing Ingredients:
- 2 green onions, chopped (optional)

Directions:
1. Preheat your oven to 350 degrees F.
2. Grease your baking pan.
3. Combine the main ingredients on the prepared sheet pan.
4. Drizzle with the oil and toss to coat.
5. Combine the seasoning ingredients in a bowl.
6. Sprinkle them over the vegetables on the pan and toss to coat with seasonings.
7. Bake in the oven for 25 minutes.

8. Stir frequently until vegetables are soft and lightly browned and chickpeas are crisp, for about 20 to 25 minutes more.
9. Season with more salt and black pepper to taste, top with the green onion before serving.

Roasted Soy Beans and Kohlrabi

Ingredients:

- 2 (15 ounce) cans soybeans, rinsed and drained
- 1/2 summer squash - peeled, seeded, and cut into 1-inch pieces
- 1 red onion, diced
- 1 large broccoli, sliced
- 2 large carrots, cut into
- 1 inch pieces
- 3 medium kohlrabi, cut into 1-inch pieces
- 3 tablespoons canola oil

Seasoning ingredients:

- 1 teaspoon salt
- 1/2 teaspoon ground black pepper
- 1 teaspoon onion powder
- 2 teaspoon garlic powder
- 1 teaspoon herbes de Provence

Garnishing Ingredients:

- 2 green onions, chopped (optional)

Directions:

1. Preheat your oven to 350 degrees F.
2. Grease your baking pan.
3. Combine the main ingredients on the prepared sheet pan.
4. Drizzle with the oil and toss to coat.
5. Combine the seasoning ingredients in a bowl.

6. Sprinkle them over the vegetables on the pan and toss to coat with seasonings.
7. Bake in the oven for 25 minutes.
8. Stir frequently until vegetables are soft and lightly browned and chickpeas are crisp, for about 20 to 25 minutes more.
9. Season with more salt and black pepper to taste, top with the green onion before serving.

Buttery Roasted Bean Sprouts & Broccoli

Ingredients:
- 1 large broccoli, sliced
- 1 cup bean sprouts
- 1 red onion, diced
- 1 sweet potato, peeled and cut into 1-inch cubes
- 2 large parsnips, cut into
- 1 inch pieces
- 3 medium potatoes, cut into 1-inch pieces
- 3 tablespoons organic salted butter

Seasoning ingredients:
- 1 teaspoon salt
- 1/2 teaspoon rainbow peppercorns
- 1 teaspoon onion powder
- 2 teaspoon garlic powder
- 1 teaspoon annatto seeds
- 1 teaspoon cumin

Garnishing Ingredients:
- 2 green onions, chopped (optional)

Directions:
1. Preheat your oven to 350 degrees F.
2. Grease your baking pan.
3. Combine the main ingredients on the prepared sheet pan.
4. Drizzle with the oil and toss to coat.

5. Combine the seasoning ingredients in a bowl.
6. Sprinkle them over the vegetables on the pan and toss to coat with seasonings.
7. Bake in the oven for 25 minutes.
8. Stir frequently until vegetables are soft and lightly browned and chickpeas are crisp, for about 20 to 25 minutes more.
9. Season with more salt and black pepper to taste, top with the green onion before serving.

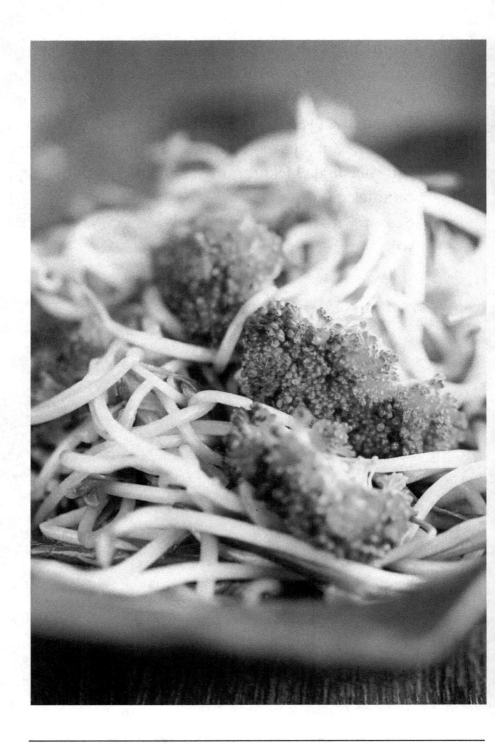

Simple and Easy Roasted Bean Sprouts and Sweet Potato

Ingredients:
- 1 large broccoli, sliced
- 1 cup bean sprouts
- 1 red onion, diced
- 1 sweet potato, peeled and cut into 1-inch cubes
- 2 large parsnips, cut into 1 inch pieces
- 3 medium potatoes, cut into 1-inch pieces
- 3 tablespoons macadamia nut oil

Seasoning ingredients:
- 1 teaspoon salt
- 1/2 teaspoon ground black pepper
- 1 teaspoon onion powder
- 2 teaspoon garlic powder
- 1/2 cup mozzarella cheese
- 1/4 cup grated parmesan cheese

Garnishing Ingredients:
- 2 green onions, chopped (optional)

Directions:
1. Preheat your oven to 350 degrees F.
2. Grease your baking pan.
3. Combine the main ingredients on the prepared sheet pan.
4. Drizzle with the oil and toss to coat.

5. Combine the seasoning ingredients in a bowl Sprinkle them over the vegetables on the pan and toss to coat with seasonings.
6. Bake in the oven for 25 minutes.
7. Stir frequently until vegetables are soft and lightly browned and chickpeas are crisp, for about 20 to 25 minutes more.
8. Season with more salt and black pepper to taste, top with the green onion before serving.

Notes

CPSIA information can be obtained
at www.ICGtesting.com
Printed in the USA
BVHW091148270521
608294BV00003B/606